Usui Tibetan Reiki Healing Energy Student Manual III

Text Copyright © 2016 Mark A. Ashford Consulting Inc.
All Rights Reserved
Paper Back ISBN: 978-1-988441-32-0
eBook ISBN: 978-1-988441-11-5

I0061550

Usui Tibetan Reiki Healing Energy Student Manual III

T his is the Student Manual for Usui Tibetan Reiki Healing Energy III. It is available as either a physical book, eBook or Audio Book. The material provides additional information and helps in exploring Reiki and is a refence for your life connection with this pure, universal energy.

There are three reasons to be attuned to Usui Tibetan Reiki Healing Energy!

1. Attuning yourself to Reiki energy has a beneficial and mindful effect on you spiritually.

2. Attunement allows you to connect to healing energy when you need it.

3. Attunement gives you the knowledge and ability to connect with healing energy not only for yourself, but others in your family and friends.

This book is designed for self-study and to support understanding of this level of Usui Tibetan Reiki healing energy.

The cost of the course includes:

1. A period of your own self-paced study.

2. A certificate of completion.

For blog posts, courses, and to book a personal remote session in Usui Tibetan Reiki Healing, or, to connect with Mark for an information session, visit Mark's website: https://www.markaashford.com and click on Contact.

Mark A. Ashford
Usui Tibetan Reiki Master and Teacher
information@markaashford.com

Usui Tibetan Reiki Healing Energy Student Manual III

1 Table of Figures

2 Introduction

As we embark on Level III Usui Reiki, let's remember that Reiki was originally developed as a system to raise one's consciousness, a spiritual science of self-development. As ever-increasing Universal Life Force - Reiki - flows through you, expect some more changes in yourself; in your thinking, your emotions, your body, your ways of interacting with the universe, its creator and with all human beings.

By asking to become a Reiki channel, a part of you, conscious or not, is stepping forward for a spiritual initiation. You're asking to develop further and a powerful opportunity is being made available to you. How you use it is of prime importance.

Our feeling is that there is not only room for many teachers, but also for many more to assist the planet and mankind through these difficult times. Learn what you can through many teachers - all of your life contacts. There are some differences in personal philosophy and abilities among teachers but there are wide differences among people too. Each teacher will draw to him or herself those that can best learn through contact with them. We bless you on your path, and thank you for sharing with us. Now let's put our heads, hands, and hearts to work.

3   Reiki - a path of empowerment

- Reiki is a very personal spiritual path/discipline which will lead to enlightenment

- Reiki is an evolutionary process that increases the natural flow of events and patterns of manifestation in life

- Reiki is a powerful tool for personal growth and transformation

- Healing is a by-product which occurs when the body is filled with this divine energy

- Remember you the physical ego self is not the healer! Reiki brings the body to its' own natural balance, allowing it to heal itself.

- Reiki reconnects the body with the holographic image of perfection or perfect light contained within its cellular structure.

- Reiki stills chaotic energy, bringing clear focus and improved concentration.

- Reiki purifies and aligns every level of your being; Breaking Down Old Patterns of Thinking, Speaking, Feeling, and Acting

- Reiki evokes the memory within that you are one with all that is. You are GOD, GOD is you. You are the earth, humanity, animals, water, air, everything that is! There is no duality or separation. Remember perfection, love, peace, truth, and the light of all this is, is you.

- When you are clear and still in mind, emotion, and body and identify with the pure light that Reiki is just by your presence, you bring into balance that which is askew and heal instantaneously. You have become Reiki pure light

- The Reiki symbols cut through or remove the veil that surrounds a person. The veil is a fog created by holding thoughts of separation negative thoughts, words, and actions.

- Each symbol tunes into a different aspect of the quality of the Reiki energy or a specific vibration. These qualities access distinctive areas of the holographic blueprint in your cellular structure.

- The breath transfers vital energy. The breath enlivens. Empower your breath and use it in all aspects of your life. Synchronize your breath with your clients for optimum benefit.

- The Attunements are sacred initiations to new levels of energy and understanding

- Reiki is an ever growing and changing energy system. It is not static. What you have learned to date is only a fraction of the fullness of Reiki. Explore the possibilities.

- Being a Reiki Master/Teacher does not mean that you are a master of Reiki; rather you've dedicated yourself to being a student of Reiki, incorporating it in every aspect of your life.

4   Reiki Purification Process

After being attuned initiated by the Reiki energy, you may be aware of an increased pace of events in your life. Time may seem to be getting shorter, with ever0increasing tasks to accomplish. Situations may seem more difficult than ever before and that may cause negative emotions to surface. What is probably happening to you is something that happens to most newly initiated Reiki practitioners; something calls a "Healing Crisis." It's purification that you are experiencing. As energy flows through the body and chakras, it is integrated, aligning and balancing every level of being. Actually, toxic remnants from past injuries, illnesses, emotional upheavals, unpleasant memories, etc., are cause physical discomforts that can last as long as 21 days.

When Reiki is purifying the physical body, flu-like symptoms may be experienced; minor discomforts including achy muscles, fever, headache, sore throat, excessive mucus, coughing, constipation, diarrhea, and other symptoms. As toxins are being released, odours in the urine and feces may change. Pressure or pains through the body, tingling, nausea or spinning sensations may also be felt in the chakras as Reiki opens, cleanses and balances them. To lessen the effects: spend extra time doing Reiki over back position #3 and over symptomatic areas. Take long walks in country settings, exercise the entire body mildly or do yoga; breathe clean, fresh air deeply into the lungs, and drink lots of pure, fresh water. Eat light nourishing meals which include fresh fruits, vegetables, and juices. A cleansing fast would also be beneficial.

 As the purification of the emotional body occurs, deeply held emotions may surface for no apparent reason; anger, frustration, grief, fear, sadness, and others. These emotions have been repressed or suppressed from earlier times in this lifetime or from past-life experiences. They are being released from the depths of your physical matrix - from the cellular level of body and mind. Do not allow yourself to become emotionally affected by what you are experiencing. Do not place blame on anyone or anything for these feelings. Just experience them as they surface and let them go.

To lessen the effects: Place one hand on your forehead and the other over your navel. Breathe in and visualize beautiful white light coming into your crown chakra, circling throughout your body and collecting all of the emotional remains; then breathe out forcefully and make a "Bah" sound, while visualizing the emotions blowing out from your solar plexus chakra. Keep this up until you feel calm. Take a long bath in dead sea salts, Epsom salts or a combination of 1 pound of sea salt and baking soda. Soak about 1/2 hour. This will relax you and help to cleanse your emotional body. Don't do this if you happen to be allergic to any of the items recommended.

When purification of the mental body occurs, old thought forms, behaviour patterns and/or habits may come to the surface. Addictive desires for food, beverages, nicotine, caffeine, alcohol, etc., may increase or resurface. Thoughts of judgment, blame, victimization, abuse, denial, self-destruction, self-pity, self-sabotage, etc., may prevail. These issues are being healed on every level of your being, from this lifetime and others. Do not be hard on yourself or allow these impulses and thoughts to get the better of you. Acknowledge them, let them go, then change your thoughts willfully to those of a more positive nature. To less the effects: Spend extra time on head positions #1, #2 and #3. Be kind to yourself. Do things that make you feel good; nurture and pamper yourself as you would a friend who was experiencing the same. Repeating positive affirmations, mantras and listening to your favourite music ease the intensity of the potentially negative effects of the thoughts.

When spiritual purification is in process, your beliefs may be shaken and challenged: beliefs in how the world operates, how relationships should be, about religion, what is important in your life, etc. As this occurs, insights, revelations, and new understanding will become clear; these will be the building blocks of your newly forming and ever-changing spiritual foundation. To lessen the effects: spend extra time doing Reiki on head positions #3 and front #1 and #2. Talk to like-minded people about your experiences, read uplifting spiritual books, listen to motivational tapes, and treat yourself with love and kindness. You are gaining new levels of understanding. During this process, you may feel lonely and perhaps fearful that you are going insane. Know that all is well and this process is perfectly normal. Be at peace. Let go and let God move through you. Continue to do Reiki on yourself; this alone can and will move you through the purification process, bringing you closer to that which you truly are; Divine spirit experiencing the physical realm of existence through the sensations of a magnificent vehicle - your body.

5   Personal Mastery Symbol

5.1   DAIKOOMYO

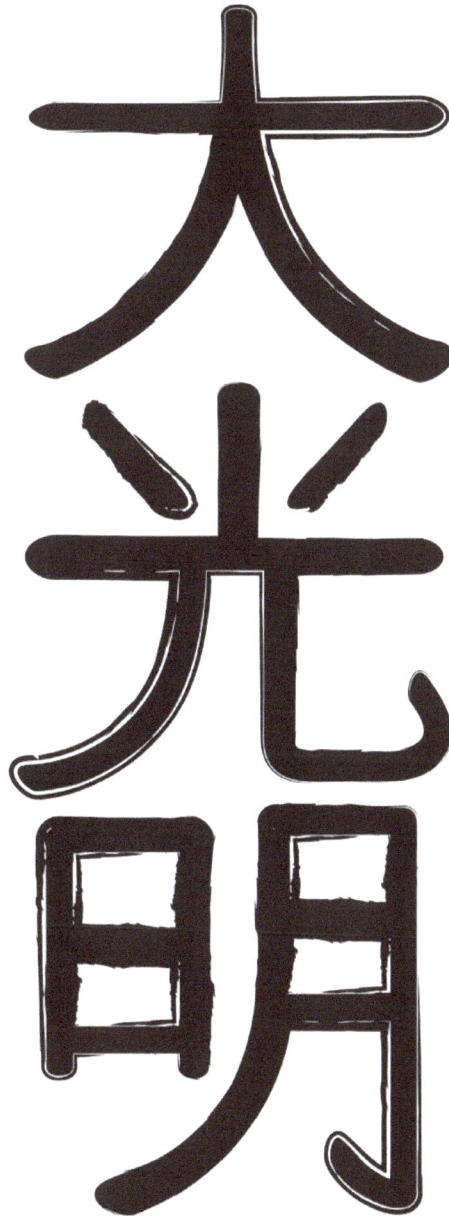

Figure 1 Reiki Symbol Daikoomyo

"Great being of the Universe, shine on me, be my friend."

The Third-Degree Symbol is the Personal Master Symbol and the meaning is

Another definition is

"The treasure-house of the great beaming light"

It represents the state of consciousness when enlightened.

Di- Big, magnificent, expansion. Large, important, dimensions

Koo- Light, radiance, or fire. Expansion at the crown chakra. Shine, beam, and brightness show one's authority and influence

Myo- Clairvoyance, clearness, discernment, open, empty, and detachment. Light piercing through the earthly planes, too clear to doubt, healing the entire world.

This symbol;

- creates a stronger connection between the physical and the higher self

- means Great Light of the Universe, enter my crown chakra and manifest through me on Earth

- is used with the other Reiki symbols

- opens crown chakra and removes veil to another dimension

- facilitates the ability of the other symbols to enter the crown and become permanently embedded in the initiate,

- brings in a higher level of Reiki during the attunement that gives the initiate a stronger, more powerful healing ability

- that always comes first; whether the client is present or in distance, healing

- increases the power of the other Reiki symbols

- intensifies and focuses. Reiki energy

- can be used to empower any kind of healing, manifesting or personal transformation work.

6   Dr. Usui's Healing Techniques

In an interview already published in Reiki, The Legacy of Dr. Usui, Dr. Usui responded to a question directly about whether his healing required any medications of any kind with the following; "It uses neither medications nor instruments. It uses only looking, blowing, stroking, light tapping, and touching of the afflicted part of the body. This is what heals diseases." The Original Reiki Handbook of Dr. Mikao Usui

One Japanese Reiki School teaches that Dr. Usui received the Reiki energy with his left hand and passed it on with his right hand. He is said to have brought the fingertips of his left hand together with the thumb as if he were holding a raw egg. The fingertips of the middle finger and ring finger of the right hand are said to have touched the tip of the right thumb. The little finger and the index finger were said to have stood away from the middle and ring finger at a ninety-degree angle. This can create a Reiki energy that can give off a laser beam of healing energy to a small area of the body. As well, by simply focusing his gaze on the area needing healing for 2 or 3 minutes, he was able to allow Reiki energy to flow into that area. The Original Reiki Handbook of Dr. Mikao Usui

7   Reiki Tapping

Standing with feet shoulder width apart, ensuring that the tip of your tongue is kept at the roof of your mouth just behind the front teeth, bending your knees slightly, placing your hands like fists on the area of your body requiring healing and lightly tapping this area while keeping an image of golden light and healing Reiki energy flowing into the affected area. The fists are turned so that the thumb is toward the ceiling and the small finger is touching area for tapping. During this time of tapping no longer than 5 minutes maximum on any area, ensure you are connecting fully with your Reiki guides and asking that they be present with you in order to remove any blockages or obstacles associated with this area and to feel a strong current of Reiki energy moving through your tapping into the area of the body.

8   The Breath

The bridge between the body and consciousness is the breath. In India it is referred to as prana, in China Chi, in Japan Ki - breath, life force energy, and Reiki. Breath is the vehicle on which energy can flow into our spiritual, emotional, mental, and physical body.

Dr. Usui taught his students a breathing technique called Joshin Kokyuu-Ho. In translation to English, this means "the breathing method for cleansing the spirit." We use this to charge ourselves with energy. Dr. Usui method is as follows;

Sit down comfortably, keeping your spine straight without becoming tense and inhale slowly through your nose. Imagine that you are breathing in not only air through your nose but also the Reiki energy through your crown chakra. Doing this breathing as a regular exercise and practice will result in a strong feeling of energy flowing through you that is readily available to you at any time.

Ensure the breath is being drawn far down into your core, directly to the energy centre two to three finger widths beneath the navel. This is known in Japan as the Tanden, in Chinese the Tantien. The Tanden is an energy centre - about the size of a grapefruit - located deep inside the Hara, roughly midway between the top of the pubic bone and the navel and is physically known as the centre of gravity.

9   The Tanden

The Tanden plays a vital role in Dr. Usui's hand positions. Taking a deep breath in and holding the breath and the energy that you have drawn in within your Tanden for a few seconds - imagine the energy from the Tanden is spreading throughout your entire body and energizing it and then slowly and deliberately exhaling through the mouth, imagining that the breath and the Reiki energy not only flow out of your mouth but also from your fingertips and the tips of your toes and out of your hand and foot chakras. This is how we become a clear channel for Reiki. The energy flows into our energy centre and then flows back through us and out into the cosmos.

Remember to ensure your tongue is on the roof of your mouth, touching your front teeth while inhaling and let it come down and rest on the bottom of the mouth while exhaling.

9.1   Storing Life Energy in the Tanden

- Concentrate the energy in your hands, fold them Gassho and imagine that you are inhaling and exhaling through your folded hands. Deepen your breathing more and more so that you are apparently inhaling through your folded hands into the Tanden and exhaling in turn. While you touch an area of the body that is negatively charged, you will feel a tingling in your hands. Let your hands rest on this area of the body until the tingling has stopped.

10   Usui Tibetan Reiki

Usui Tibetan Reiki is the name given to the system that was developed by Arthur Robertson in our lineage, which was later made popular and well known through William Lee Rand and Diane Stein. This system is derived from Usui Reiki, as taught by Takata, and includes all healing techniques of Dr. Usui as well as some additions; a modified attunement method that incorporates the Violet breath, the use of the Usui Tibetan master and Kundalini fire symbols along with the four traditional Usui symbols: the Hui yin position and also the microcosmic orbit. Usui Tibetan Reiki can sometimes incorporate psychic surgery or etheric cleansing.

11   Tibetan Symbols

11.1   Tibetan Master Symbol – Dumo

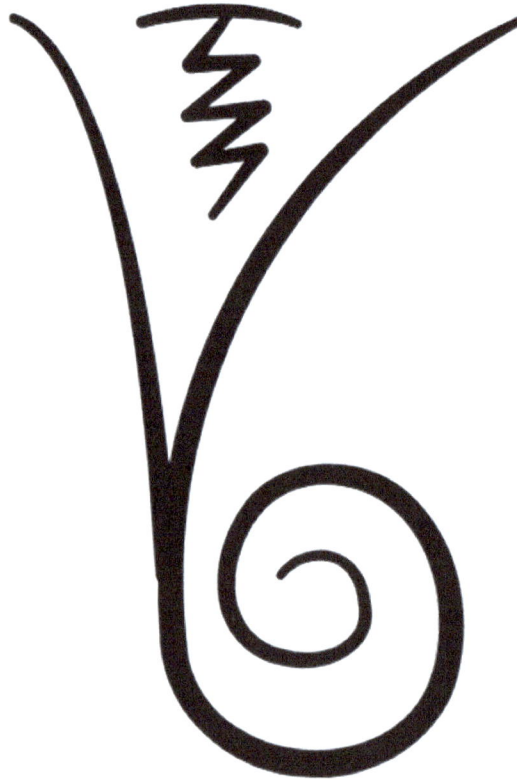

Figure 2 Reiki Symbol Dumo

Represents the swirling fiery heat of the Kundalini. Dumo or Dumo fire is the heat which ascends over the spine as a result of Kundalini awakening. The unification of mind and body produces the emanation of heat. Heat is the lowest range of vibrations, radiating out to produce form body. Also, sometimes called Motor / Zanon.

- Dumo is the igniter of the sacred flame or Kundalini fire. As Kundalini is awakened and ascends the central channel, it revitalizes and energizes the centre of each chakra, purifying the astral channels related to each of the chakras.

- Unifies the mind and body

- works with the fire in the base chakra

- It rapidly travels from the healer's brain/hand to the area of the receiver's body where it is most needed

- Reversing the spiral in a counterclockwise direction, inner Ki expands to connect with Ki beyond the body. When the expansion is complete, the direction automatically reverses, bringing Ki within. A spiral creates a vortex that intensifies the energy.

- It pulls negative energy and disease out of the body and releases it.

- It heals the soul

- can be used on crystals, asking the stones to self-clear henceforth and forever

- Use when making flower or gem elixirs; add Dumo Symbol and Power Symbol to the water while they are infusing in the sun

- Its focus is healing

- Can also be used in the attunement process with Violet Breath.

12   Tibetan Fire Serpent

The Tibetan Fire Serpent represents the Serpent Kundalini Power coiling at the base of the spine. Also known as Fire Dragon

- use during attunement with horizontal line over the top of the crown, snaking down the spine and spiralling at the base of the spine; ground energy into the body.

- Reversing the spiral clockwise starting at the base of the spine, snaking up the spine, ending with horizontal line over crown, can bring on Kundalini experience.

- Connects and opens all chakras.

- Opens central channel allowing the flow of Kundalini fire.

- Can be used in healing or meditation for more balance and receptivity. Draw or visualize purple or gold, with horizontal line overhead, wavy line going down connecting all chakras and spiral ending at base chakra.

13   Kundalini Energy

Kundalini[1] is energy. It is dormant at the bottom of the spine, in the root chakra until awakened. It has been there since birth as one of the gifts people receive.

Kundalini awakening offers a profound opportunity for those called to follow a spiritual path. It gradually releases many patterns, conditions, and delusions of the separate self. It can be threatening to the ego-structure because a person may feel a loss of interest in their old life and identity, and consciousness may go into unfamiliar expansive or empty states that are disorienting. It also makes people who are unfamiliar with it afraid they are ill or losing their minds. So, understanding it is important.[2]

Once awakened, it travels up the central Nadi – also called Sushumna. Alongside or inside the spine, it depends on the awakening and the individual. As it travels, the energy flows through each chakra, generating various levels of mystical experience for the individual. When it reaches the Crown Chakra, a change in consciousness, some say a profound change, takes place. The awakened person may use the brain to transmute the energy into the highest form of energy called 'Ojas.'

Dumo is the Tibetan Master Symbol. It represents the swirling fiery heat of the Kundalini. Dumo or Dumo fire is the heat which ascends over the spine as a result of Kundalini awakening. The

---

[1] "Kundalini," *Wikipedia*, September 8, 2018, https://en.wikipedia.org/w/index.php?title=Kundalini&oldid=858570525.
[2] "What Is Kundalini?," The Kundalini Guide, accessed September 15, 2018, http://www.kundaliniguide.com/what-is-kundalini/.

unification of mind and body produces the emanation of heat. Heat is the lowest range of vibrations, radiating out to produce form or body.

It ignites the sacred flame or Kundalini fire. As Kundalini is awakened and ascends the central channel, it revitalizes and energizes the centre of each chakra, purifying the astral channels related to each of the chakras.

Dumo unifies the mind and body and works with the fire in the base chakra. It rapidly travels from the healer's brain/hand to the area of the receiver's body where it is most needed.

Reversing the spiral in the Dumo Fire symbol to clockwise direction, starting at the base, inner Ki expands to connect with Ki beyond the body. When the expansion is complete, the direction automatically reverses, bringing Ki within. A spiral creates a vortex that intensifies the energy. It pulls negative energy and disease out of the body and releases it and heals the soul.

It can be used on crystals, asking the stones to self-clear henceforth and forever

Use when making flower or gem elixirs; add Dumo Symbol and Power Symbol to the water while they are infusing in the sun

Its focus is healing

Can also be used in the attunement process with Violet Breath.

14 RAKU

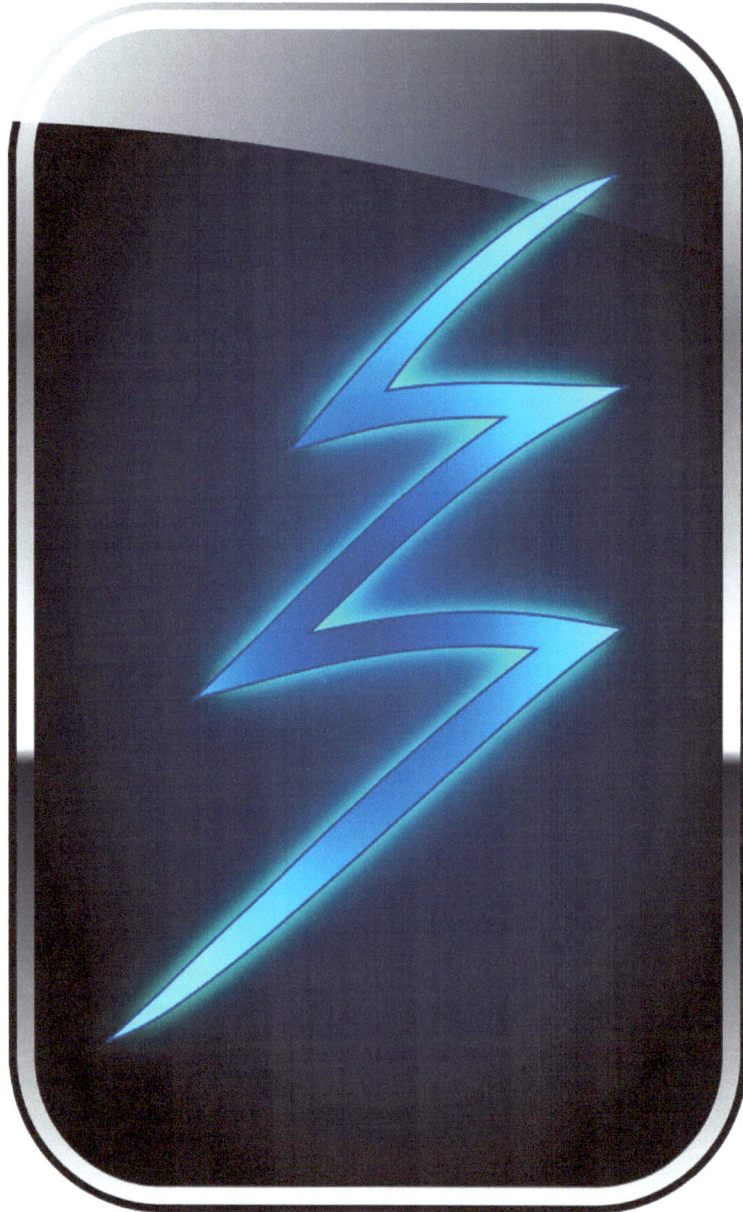

Figure 3 Reiki Symbol Raku

The raku is represented by the Lightning Bolt and is defined as 'banking the fire."

- Used in passing Attunements but not in healing

- Used in the beginning of an attunement, it helps to lift negative karma and takes initiate to higher levels of consciousness.

- At the end of an attunement, it separates the auras of the Master and student.

- Use the symbol from feet to crown to take a person out of the body, and from crown to feet for grounding and to draw the energy from the universe into the body.

14.1 Ran Sei

pronounced Lan Say

Inflammation

- A healing symbol

- is used to clear infection and reduce inflammation.

14.2 Ren So Mai

pronounced   Len So My

Angelic energies

- Brings feelings of unconditional love

- Use in attunement process at heart and sweep off hands

- Used to bring in angelic energies

    1.

15   The Hara

Hara located between the navel and the pelvis literally speaks to the stomach and abdomen and includes the digestion, absorption, and elimination functions of the physical body. The Hara also includes the solar plexus physical location and also some of its spiritual and energetic significance. It is a driving force of psychic energy, simply meaning that it contains energy here that cannot be contributed either physiologically or psychologically. Harada-Roshi, a celebrated Zen master, encouraged his students to focus all of their attention on their Hara and would say, "You must realize that the centre of the universe is the pit of your belly!"

It is frequently referred to as "The Seat of Enlightenment." The more energy and attention that are directed toward this area, a body/mind equilibrium shifts, ensuring a focus of vital energy that continues to strengthen and among other things, alleviates mental clutter and confusion from the brain and promotes clarity, emotional stability, and groundedness in thinking. Physical effects can be a loosening of the neck and shoulder muscles, better posture, and deeper breathing as well as a new sense of emotional and spiritual freedom.

16   Contacting the Hui Yin

Contacting the Hui Yin and the Violet Breath are done during the Usui Reiki attunements and can be done with other attunement methods as well. If you practise them on a regular basis, you will experience a sense of well0being. Physical and emotional problems will begin to clear and endorphins in the brain will cause a natural high, leading to increased spiritual awareness and a well-developed body-mind-spirit connection.

The Hui Yin is an acupuncture point located at the perineum, between the rectum and the genitals. With the continuous muscle contracting of the Hui Yin point and increased amount of high frequency, chi enters your system and passes through the Hui Yin point during the attunement process.

For women: Learning to contract the Hui Yin connects the functional/Conception and governing channels at the top and bottom of the body, allowing Ki to move in a complete circuit. The closing of the Hui Yin brings Earthly Ki upward into the Hara while at the same time drawing Heavenly Ki downward to the Hara as well. This exercise teaches one to do the contraction with external pressure, allowing the Master/Teacher to move around while passing Reiki attunements. While holding the Hui Yin, place your tongue on the roof of your mouth, in the groove behind the teeth. This closes the energy circuit between the Conception and governing channels. The Ki moves from the crown downward, from the Earth upward and the Hara is activated.

16.1   For Men:

This exercise is the same for men as for women, with one exception; only the anus in contracted. Draw the muscles up and in, closing the two gates where sexual energy is lost. With the anus contracted, the Ki immediately moves upward along the Hara line. Earth's energy is then drawn into the Hara. While holding the Hui Yin, place your tongue on the roof of your mouth, in the groove behind the teeth. This closes the energy circuit between the Conception and governing channels. The Ki moves from the crown downward, from the Earth upward and the Hara is activated.

17   Violet Breath

1. Contract the Hui Yin point, place your tongue to the roof of your mouth.

2. Draw in a breath, imagining it as a white light coming down through the Crown Chakra, through the tongue, down the front of the body through the Hui Yin point and up the spine, filling the centre of the head.

3. Visualize the while light turning blue and rotating clockwise, they turn violet.

4. Within the violet light, picture a golden Personal Mastery Symbol

5. Exhale gently into initiate's Crown Chakra, imagine personal mastery symbol on your breath entering into initiate's head and lodging in the Heart Chakra or to the base of the brain for initiatory attunements; say sacred name 3 times.

18   Etheric Cleansing

The cause of most diseases is an accumulation of negative psychic energy, which is usually composed of negative thoughts and feelings that block the flow of life force. This non-physical negative energy forms into clumps with a particular shape and lodges itself in or around the physical organs, chakras or in the aura, and can be removed using this technique.

This tool can be used to facilitate the healing of any issue, including physical health problems, career and money problems, emotional difficulties, relationships, addictions, mental imbalances, spiritual problems, etc.

Etheric surgery can be used in conjunction with a regular Reiki treatment. Start with a healing attunement, followed by psychic surgery and then a full-Reiki treatment.

To find the location of the energy block:

1. Ask the client to describe the problem to be healed

2. Ask them to close their eyes and meditate on the problem. Say, "If this problem existed in your body, where would it manifest?" There are no wrong answers.

3. Tell them to look into the area and ask, "If this problem had a shape, what would it look like?" It's important that the client describe the negative energy and not internal organs.

4. Repeat the same procedure with colour, texture, weight, and sound so they have a clear image of the negative energy, as a real object.

5. Have them focus on the shape and meditate on letting go of it. Ask if they are willing to learn any lessons or receive any information related to the healing process.

18.1   The Cleansing procedure

1. The client can be standing, sitting or lying down.

2. Draw the personal Mastery symbol on both of your hands, say name 3 times, and clap hands 3 times. Repeat with the Power Symbol. Draw a large power symbol down the front of your body for protection and over each of your chakras to open them, saying name 3 times at each position.

3. Pull on your physical fingers and imagine extending them out 6-8 inches. While pulling, make a stretching sound by breathing in through partly closed lips so you can hear air flowing. Repeat 3 times. Pat the ends of your extended fingers and imagine you can feel them. Draw the Power Symbol on the ends of the fingers of both hands.

4. Invoke the guidance and assistance from your Reiki guides, asking that divine love and wisdom direct the healing for the highest good of all concerned.

5. Draw the Power Symbol over the area to be worked on.

6. Using the full strength of your total being, imagine you are reaching in, grabbing the negative energy with your extended Reiki fingers, pulling it out and sending it up to the light.

7. As you reach in to grab the negative energy, breath in through partly closed lips audibly, absorbing the energy block into your fingers; release same energy upward toward the light, vigorously blowing the breath out. This will prevent the negative energy from entering your body.

8. Repeat this procedure for several minutes, allowing your higher intuition to guide you on how to proceed.

9. Periodically, ask the client if he/she feels any change; continuing to work until the negative energy is no longer felt.

10. If negative energy persists, lace your hands on the area, mentally draw the mental/emotional symbol and ask for guidance from it; what lesson needs to be learned, or what it needs to heal. The intuitive input of both you and the client is important.

11. Use the guidance that comes. Sometimes, healing may be accomplished in the session; other times, it may happen after the session. Continue with additional psychic cleansing surgery asking the client to report the results. Occasionally, a process of release begins that continues for several hours or days.

12. Afterwards, fill the area with Reiki energy. Use the Power Symbol to seal the treatment

13. 'karate chop' the air between you and the client to break the energy connection. Retract your Reiki fingers back as you make a noise with the breath. Rinse off hands in cold water to elbows.

14. Finish with a full Reiki treatment using all the hand positions.

19   Microcosmic Orbit in Reiki

"Ki" of Reiki is the life force energy, called Prana, means "breath" or "a body of energy acting as the medium for carrying consciousness" - the animating force of Be-Ing. It is the connecting link between the physical, energy, and spirit bodies.

Earthly and Heavenly Ki are drawn into the body from without. Original Ki is inward and is stored in the space between the navel and belly chakra, called the Hara. The Ki flows and circulates through the body via energy channels.

There are three main channels running vertically through the body, called Kundalini. The great central channel runs along the spinal column from crown to root, called the "Sushumna" Hara Line, and is the connection between the energies of Earth and the universe; its charge is neutral.

The pairs of opposite moving channels are the "Ida" and "Pingala" moving in an intertwining path along the Sushumna. Pingala begins at perineum Hui Yin, is masculine and rises upward along the spine. Governor or governing vessel/Channel, while Ida begins at crown, is feminine and has downward movement on the front of the body. Conception or Functional Vessel/Channel

The microcosmic orbit predates Reiki and is from Taoist practice. It is completed and practised to enhance vitality and health. When this practice is held through a Reiki session by a Reiki practitioner, it increases the ability to channel Reiki energy and can provide clearer guidance and awareness for the healer.

Branching from these primary channels are all of the large and small acupuncture lines called the "Meridians" and "Nadi's."

20 Sushumna

Sushumna Nadi is the central channel of energy in the human body that runs from the base of the spine. It is situated at the perineum, which is also known as Muladhara or Root Chakra too.

Brahmadanda, which anatomically coincides with what is known as the fourth ventricle, is the place where the cerebrum spinal fluid governs transmittance of all. The area incorporates the hypothalamus, pineal and pituitary glands. This is the Sahaswara or Crown chakra of the head and carries Kundalini energy, the primal evolutionary force within and upward as it is awakened through the practice of yoga and meditation.

Sushumna Nadi only opens and flows freely when Ida and Pingala nadis are balanced and clear; thus, the purification of all three nadis is important for the overall health and wellness of the body and mind, and one can also experience spiritual growth.

Sushumna: Passes through the spinal column, connecting the 1st root chakra to the 7th crown chakra. Sushumna is the path through which Kundalini shakti, and the higher spiritual consciousness it can fuel, rise up from its origin in the first chakra to its true home at the 7th chakra. In yoga and other traditions, the Sushumna Nadi is thus the path to enlightenment. [3]

Ida: Spirals around the Sushumna Nadi, beginning and ending on the left of it, crossing with Pingala at each chakra. Carrier of lunar, female energy. Cool and nurturing, controls mental processes and the more feminine aspects of our personality. Nourishes and purifies the body and the mind. [4]

Pingala: Spirals around the Sushumna Nadi, beginning and ending to the right of it, crossing with Ida at each chakra. Warm and stimulating, controls vital physical processes, and oversees the more masculine aspects of our personality. Carrier of solar, male energy, adding vitality, physical strength and efficiency. [5]

Anahata said, "However, as a spiritualist, even though I personally enjoy all the technicalities of ancient wisdom and esoteric arts, I don't obsess over them. If our spiritual urge or intent is aligned with infinite expansion of awareness, potentials, and consciousness, to love, to higher principles of freedom and balance for the highest good of all, then any sincere spiritual practice, be it yoga or plant spirit medicine, drum medicine or reiki, should support this process effectively.

---

[3] "Acupuncture Meridians and Nadis: Basics About Acupressure's Energy Channels," The Energy Healing Site, accessed September 26, 2018, https://www.the-energy-healing-site.com/acupuncture-meridians.html.
[4] "Acupuncture Meridians and Nadis."
[5] "Acupuncture Meridians and Nadis."

20.1 The Microcosmic Orbit

The microcosmic orbit is a vital part of the Reiki attunement process. It connects the Conception and the governing vessel channels to make a completed energy circle throughout the body.

The history of the microcosmic orbit dates back to prehistoric times in China, and the underlying principles can be found in the I Ching, which, according to legend, was written by the Emperor Fu Xi approximately five thousand years ago or at least two centuries before the time of the Yellow Emperor. [6]

The Microcosmic Orbit 小周天, also known as the 'Self-Winding Wheel of the Law' and the circulation of light, is a Taoist Qigong or Taoist yoga Ki energy cultivation technique. It involves deep breathing exercises in conjunction with meditation and concentration techniques, which develop the flow of ki along certain pathways of energy in the human body, which may be familiar to those who are studying traditional Chinese medicine, qigong, T'ai chi ch'uan, Neidan and Taoist alchemy. [7]

The first step is to connect the channels at the Root Chakra by closing the Hui Yin position, forcing energy to move upward along the spine. The second step connects the channels at the top of the body by placing the tongue on the roof of the mouth behind the teeth. The reason for doing the exercises is to receive and channel greater amounts of Ki energy, giving you the ability to pass Reiki Attunements to initiates more effectively. Your Reiki healing treatments and Attunements will also become more powerful when you incorporate the microcosmic orbit while doing a hands-on treatment.

_____

[6] "Microcosmic Orbit," _Wikipedia_, January 29, 2018,
https://en.wikipedia.org/w/index.php?title=Microcosmic_orbit&oldid=822922386.
[7] "Microcosmic Orbit."

21 Meditation

21.1 Microcosmic Orbit Meditation - Small Heavenly Cycle

Does the microcosmic orbit while meditating with energy focused inward?

1. Begin by visualizing a Power Symbol at your Hara point halfway between navel and pubic bone

2. When warmth Ki is felt, move it by intent to the perineum Hui Yin point

3. Now direct it up the spine to the top of the head pineal gland. Crown chakra. Hold this visualization/energy for up to ten minutes. Continue to see the Power Symbol moving up the spine.

4. Direct it by intent downward to the upper lip. Touch the roof of the mouth just behind the teeth with the tongue, allowing the power symbol/energy to continue flowing down the front of the body to regather at the Hara.

5. Hold at the Hara until the warmth collects again, then start the orbit again.

6. Repeat the circle several times. Increase with practice to thirty-six orbits per session.

21.2 Great Heavenly Cycle - Earth Exercise

After you become proficient with the above, include the following Earth exercise.

1. From the navel, direct the power symbol/energy flow to the Hui Yin, then divide it into two channels, sending power symbols and ki down the back of the thighs, past the knees and calves to the soles of the feet. The K-1 points Yung-Chuan on both soles is the body's electrical connection Earth chakra with the Earth's energy.

2. Once the warmth builds in the soles, move the power symbol/energy to the big toes, up the tops of the feet, past the knees, up the insides of the thighs and back to the Hui Yin.

3. Continue to draw energy from the Earth through the soles throughout this exercise.

4. Return the power symbol/energy flow up the spine Governing Channel and divide it again at the T-5/T-6 point between the shoulder blades Gia Pe

5. Concentrate on feeling energy accumulates, then direct the power symbol/energy along the middle fingers, over the backs of the hands, up the outside of the arms, over the shoulders and reconnecting at the spine.

6. Continuing up the neck past the Crown and down the front Conception Channel to the Hara.

7. Repeat several times, stopping at following locations to visualize the Power Symbol and allow the feeling of the Ki energy to accumulate, then move on; Hara, Hui Yin, K-1 on soles, Hui Yin,

Kidney point Ming-Men, on spine opposite navel, Thymus Chakra Gia Pe, point opposite heart, Jade Pillow Yu-Chen, cranial pump at the base of the skull, pineal gland at Crown, Pai Hui, Third eye between brows, heart, Hara.

IMPORTANT: Complete the microcosmic orbit meditation by grounding it, after one energy circuit or many. With the energy at the Hara, place your fist lightly over your navel and rub in a spiral no more than 6 inches wide motion; women - spiral counterclockwise thirty-six times, then clockwise twenty-four times men the opposite. This prevents electrical overload and discomfort.

22   Usui Tibetan Reiki Healing Energy - Attunement

The healing attunement is for personal growth and expanded awareness. You now become a co-creator of Energy. Attunements access your inner wholeness or light seed; your God self. It will open you to higher energies and put your consciousness in the dynamic process of multidimensional access.

The healing attunement centres and balances the body. Do it on yourself or others every day; as often as possible. Some people do as many as 50-60 Attunements a day. Send Attunements with each position during absentee treatments. Attunements are not just for crisis situations. Incorporate them into your daily activities. [8]

Attunement is a form of energy medicine originally developed by Lloyd Arthur Meeker 1907 – 1954 and his colleagues. Meeker taught and practiced attunement as a central feature of his spiritual teaching and ministry, Emissaries of Divine Light. Attunement is taught as a personal spiritual practice and as a healing modality offered through the hands. Emissaries of Divine Light believe that attunement is a pivotal factor in the conscious evolution of humanity.

22.1   HEALING ATTUNEMENT - Non-Reiki and First-Degree

This attunement will open and bring in higher energy, raise vibrations, release negativity and re-establish balance.

2. Invite people to sit in a chair. Make sure you have enough room to walk around chair. Say to them, "Please keep your feet flat on the floor, hands in prayer position at heart, legs uncrossed, and eyes closed until I tell you to open them."

3. Imagine a circle of light, 3 feet in all directions, around the person. Consider this a sacred space.

4. Call upon your guides, masters, and teachers to guide and assist you during this healing Attunement.

5. Contract the Hui Yin, touch tongue to the roof of the mouth and hold throughout attunement feel energy building at Hara

6. Put your left hand straight up in the air, palm facing forward. With your right-hand draw in front of you all four symbols Daikumyo, Hunshazishuneen, Sei He Ki, and Chokurey - say each name 3 times. This brings energy into the person doing the attunement; prepares and protects the space in the room.

---

[8] Beacons of Change, "Reiki Attunement," (2025).

7. Step into the circle of light, moving to the right, until you are behind the person. Don't step out of the circle or you must start over.

8. Hold breath, visualizing energy building in Hara.

9. Extend your left arm straight up, palm flat, facing forward. With your right-hand flat over the crown, draw using entire hand the Personal Mastery Symbol curving symbol around head ending at the base of the skull; say name 3 times. Above crown chakra, draw the Power Symbol, and say name 3 times. Lightly rest right hand on crown chakra. Mentally draw or visualize the distance, Mental/Emotional and Power symbols, say each name 3 times. Bring your hands into prayer position.

10. Release breath into crown.

11. Coming around to the front, walking around to the right - do not step out of the circle and always face the receiver of the attunement.

12. With your left hand, place the thumb and forefinger on the centre of the backs of their hands. Lightly touch your right-hand finger tips to their fingertips; three middle fingers touching the thumb and little finger pointing to their thumb and little finger. Mentally draw or visualize all 4 symbols, say each name 3 times. Visualize placing these symbols in their hands.

13. Place your left hand over your heart, right hand above their right shoulder at head level. Move your hand to their forehead, then down to the base of the spine, draw 3 spirals up from base to third eye last spiral circles. Hands. Place your right hand lightly over their heart chakra and say mentally, "As above, so below."

14. Place your left-hand thumb and forefinger on the centre of the backs of their hands, right-hand fingers cupping over their fingertips. Mentally draw or visualize all 4 symbols, say each name 3 times.

15. Draw in and hold breath, visualizing energy building at Hara.

16. Place your finger slightly on their wrists and align their fingertips with their third eye. Exhale breath in 3 puffs - first, through finger tips to third eye - second, through the base of hands to heart - third, through finger tips to crown. Separate and place their hands on their hearts.

17. Place your hands on your heart; take at least 3 steps backward until you are out of the sacred space.

18. Align your left hand in front middle of your face, finger tips at third eye. With the right hand, draw the Power Symbol, starting from above the right shoulder; move to forehead; down to base of spine; spiral up to third eye third spiral circles your hand say name 3 times; place right hand on your heart; say mentally, "As above, so below."

19. Draw in and hold breath, visualizing energy building at Hara.

20. Bring hands into prayer position. Imagine a mirror in front of you; exhale in 3 puffs, through finger tips to your third eye, through the base of the hand to your heart, then through finger tips to Crown.

21. Thank and bow to your guides, Masters, and helpers.

22. Ask the person to take a deep breath and open their eyes when they are ready; wait for eye contact; bow to them.

When attunement is completed, do not ask the person what they have experienced. They will share if they want to.

22.2 HEALING ATTUNEMENT FOR SECOND DEGREE AND ABOVE

Before you give the attunement, ask which is their dominant hand.

1. Follow steps 1 through 12 above.

2. Draw in and hold breath, visualizing energy building at Hara

3. Place their non-dominant hand over their heart. Take their dominant hand, palm up into your left hand. With your right hand, draw the Power symbol over their open palm; say name 3 times. Blow in open palm; then lightly slap palm 3 times and hold for a few seconds.

4. Draw in and hold breath, visualizing energy building at Hara.

5. Place their dominant hand over their heart. Take their non-dominant hand, palm up, into your left hand. With your right hand, draw the Power symbol over their open palm; say name 3 times. Blow on open palm, then lightly slap palm 3 times and hold for a few seconds.

6. Bring both of their hands back into prayer position.

22.3 SELF-Attunement

1. Sit or stand legs uncrossed

2. Ask for guidance and assistance from masters and guides. Mentally visualize a circle of light around yourself.

3. Contract Hui Yin, touch tongue to roof of mouth hold throughout attunement

4. Draw in and hold breath, visualizing energy building at Hara.

5. Hold left arm straight above head, palm facing forward. With the right hand, draw the Personal Mastery Symbol; say name 3 times. Draw the power symbol flat over crown; say name 3 times. Rest right hand lightly on Crown. Mentally draw or visualize the distance, Mental/Emotional and Power symbols, say names 3 times.

6. Release breath, visualizing it entering down.

7. Align left hand in half prayer position; finger tips at third eye. Place right-hand finger tips to the finger tips of the left hand. Mentally draw or visualize all 4 symbols over hands; say each name 3 times. Draw a three-dimensional power symbol, starting at right of shoulder, move to forehead; down to base; spiral up to third eye third spiral circles your hand say name 3 times; place right hand on your heart; say mentally, "As above, so below"

8. cup right-hand fingers over left finger tips. Mentally draw or visualize all 4 symbols over hands; say each name 3 times.

9. Draw In and Hold Breath, Visualizing Energy Building at Hara

10. Bring hands together in prayer position. Imagine a mirror in front of you; blow 3 puffs, through finger tips to third eye; under palms to heart; over finger tips to crown. Place your hands on your heart for a moment.

11. Bring hands into prayer position; thank and bow to your guides, Masters, and helpers.

12. Take a deep breath and open your eyes when you are ready.

22.4 Expansion Healing Attunement

Expands awareness of energy beyond physical body and senses

1. For Self: Same steps as "Self-Attunement," but without touching the body. Hold your right hand about an inch above your head and hands.

2. For others: Same steps as "Healing Attunement," but without touching the body. Hold your hands about an inch above their head and hands to move their hands lightly lift and guide them with your forefingers.

22.5 Absentee Healing Attunement

1. Use a picture of people to be attuned; empower with Second Degree techniques to represent the person

2. Place picture on chair

3. Follow steps 2 through 20 of HEALING ATTUNEMENT. When doing their hands, use your left hand in half-prayer position and your right hand for 'finger tips to finger tips' and for 'cupping.' For 3-dimensional power symbol, use your left hand in half prayer position; move right hand from above where their right shoulder would be; to forehead; down to the base of the spine. Draw 2 spirals up from base to third eye. The last spiral circles your hand. Place your right hand where their heart would be; say mentally, "As above, so below." When doing the breath, blow across your hands to where the person's third eye, heart, and crown would be.

23 Additional Information About Attunements

- When there is not a picture available, write a person's name on paper, empower with all symbols; follow steps in "Absentee Healing Attunement." Attunement can be done in this way also for events, situations, pets, earth, relationships, etc.

- For hospital patients, treat as above, mentally walking behind patient; Even Through Walls

- Do attunement mentally to time yourself while doing hands-on or absentee treatments. An attunement takes approximately 5 minutes.

- Always remember to use two sets of breaths when doing absentee attunements.

- Send attunements to the planet, guides, Angels, Masters, events, situations, etc.

- Reiki and healing attunements are not just for times of illness or imbalance.

23.1 Mental/Emotional Attunement

To increase the effectiveness of the mental/emotional balancing techniques you learned in the second degree, add the following attunement.

1. With your dominant hand, draw the mental/emotional and the power symbols on the head; inhale drawing the power symbol with tongue on the roof of the mouth and breathe on the head breath brings life to symbols.

Add this to the mental/emotional techniques to use it alone during a regular hands-on treatment.

23.2 Temporarily Attuning Hands to Do Reiki

For People Who Are Not Attuned to Any Level of Reiki

You can temporarily attune someone's hands to do Reiki during a group treatment.

1. Visualize all 4 symbols in the person's hands, say names 3 times, say "By the Law of Correspondence, this person's hands represent my hands during this Reiki session" specify length of time.

The person's hands will channel Reiki during the time period you a lot, and can last as long as 24 hours after the attunement.

24 Meditation

24.1 Manifesting Goals

This is a very powerful meditation that combines the advantages of other types plus the healing power of the Reiki energies. It is physically relaxing, bringing mental clarity, improved visualization, clairvoyance, enhanced healing skills and expansion of consciousness. It can also be used to solve problems and goals. The more you practise the technique, the more it increases in value.

1. Find a comfortable position, with your hands resting on your legs or any relaxing position. Close your eyes and breathe slowly and deeply.

    2. Using your whole hand, draw and visualize the personal Mastery symbol in the air in front of your eyes. Say its name 3 times aloud, if alone, otherwise silently. Hold the image for up to 15 minutes then imagine it moving up into a field of light above you. Bring your attention back in front of your eyes.

    3. Repeat step #2 with each of the other symbols; The Power, Mental / Emotional and Distance Symbols

    4. After meditating on each symbol for a while, you will be centred and highly charged with creative, healing energies that you may use to work on projects, actualize goals, send help or healing to others at a distance.

24.2 Using Meditation to Manifest Goals

1. State your goal out loud or silently to yourself; visualize completed goal and mentally surround it with the four Reiki symbols. Hold this image until you have a feeling of accomplishment. Do this for each project, goal, or healing treatment sent then state; "If this is possible within divine love and wisdom, then let it be so." Lastly, with a feeling of fulfillment, send the image completed goal and surrounding Reiki symbols up into a field of light.

2. To finish the meditation, place your tongue to the roof of your mouth and focus on the area just behind your navel. Draw the Power Symbol down the front of your body, with spiral circling navel say the name 3 times and hold attention on this spot for up to 10 minutes. This will release any excess build-up of head energy and store in your power centre.

3. Continuing to breathe slowly; open your eyes, and take some time to journal your experiences.

If you have difficulty visualizing, write out the goal or healing on a piece of paper along with the four Reiki symbols. State that it has been achieved; surround it with light and completely release it from your conscious attention.

25   Crystal Healing

This type of healing works on two levels; the way in which our body or mind responds to the energy being emitted from each crystal and also the way in which we perceive and believe the healing can and will take place. All good health is a balance between the physical, emotional, and mental states. Any crystals can be useful for balancing energies whether placed in the hand, around the room or on the recipient's body over an area that requires healing or over each of the 7 main chakra points.

By using your intuition, you can experiment by choosing different types of crystals to wear or carry with you throughout the day and notice the difference in your energy, awareness, and overall wellness of spirit as you continue to carry this crystal with you, generally approx. Three days is appropriate to begin to notice a benefit. Notice which types of crystals you are drawn to and make note of the properties they hold understanding why you were drawn here and what part of your spirit emotionally, physically and/or spiritually you may be requiring some additional healing frequencies from this particular crystal.

25.1   How Crystals Affect Our Energy

Our own life force energy called chi in Chinese medicine and prana in Indian medicine moves within us as subtle energy, which is an entire network of energy through which, when undisturbed, feelings such as joy, happiness, love, compassion, and well-being flow freely also. This subtle body can be disturbed through fear and other negative mental states and then this energy becomes restricted and can cause anxiety, fear, depression, etc. Our chi travels around on energy pathways within our body, known as meridians and our body contains 12 of them. As well, there are 7 major energy centres known as chakras within and as we line up our crystals over these chakra points and meridian lines as we are guided…we can benefit from a rebalancing of our energy - clearing out blockages and restoring our flow of chi/prana/life force energy.

25.2   Balancing Energy With Crystals

To balance your energy is to find a balance between yin feminine and yang masculine, which is a balance between positive and negative attributes. e.g., if you are feeling joyful, then your ability to feel depressed is very low or if you are feeling fearful, then your opposing feeling of peace is very low and therefore finding a balance between the two can greatly assist in being able to moderate your energy and balance optimal health.

When balancing energy, the personality of the person should be considered. Dr. Meyer Friedman, an American Cardiologist, and his colleague Dr. R. H. Rosenman, developed the theory of personality types. For example, Type A personalities are chronically angry and impatient people raise their risk of heart attacks. Type B personality types are mellower, and have a more thoughtful behaviour. The personality type affects the person's health and ability to deal with stress and as cardiologists, they considered the personality type as having an effect on heart health. [9]

The following crystals are associated with type a personalities:

- Rutilated quartz

- Obsidian

- Smokey Quartz

- Crysocolla

- Malachite

- Purple fluorite

- Clear quartz

Calming crystals are:

- Amethyst

- Rose quartz

---

[9] "Meyer Friedman," *Wikipedia*, September 12, 2018, https://en.wikipedia.org/w/index.php?title=Meyer_Friedman&oldid=859248499.

26   How to Heal with Crystals

Crystals can interact with your own bioelectric energy field and while the crystal itself does very little, if anything, to positively or negatively affect a person, place or thing - the relationship with another energy source can be a powerful source of healing. Crystals have the ability to hold positive healing energy and emit healing frequencies and vibrations that can positively affect situations in which they are being held or even situations where the healer is intending their healing properties to be sent to distantly.

26.1   Energy Charge / Activating Your Crystals

This converts pressure into an electrical charge. Using your breath to charge the crystal energetically, the energy loops from the crystal back to you until a maximum energy charge is reached. Now the energy can be discharged from the crystal and as directed by the crystal holder's intent or thought patterns.

26.2   Penetrating Healing Energy

Crystal energy can transmit through any substance, such as layers of clothing, skin, etc. When crystals are placed on the body, the healing properties of the crystal together with the healing intent of the healer are transmitted to the recipient.

26.3   Projected healing energy

Crystals can be used in a similar manner for distance healing, like in a distant Reiki healing session. Energy can be sent and received when these crystals act as conductors for healing energy over short distances and even globally in this manner.

26.4   Programming your Crystal

While each and every crystal has it owns task/preprogrammed energy, each crystal also comes with its own bland database, which has the ability to store new instructions or absorb its healers intent. The crystal can translate and absorb an energy signature and work it in with its own crystalline energy structure, which can then be used later for healing.

26.5   Attuning Yourself to Your Crystals

This is a process that aligns your energy to that of your crystal. Holding a clear quartz crystal in your right hand and drawing a circle about 1" above over your left palm and then vice versa. Also run clockwise circles in the same manner over your heart chakra, feeling the electrical charge both in your palms and also within and around your heart chakra, repeating an alignment verse that may be as follows or one that resonates with you, "I dedicate this crystal to healing and to universal energy. It is my intention to work together with this crystal's healing properties and energies for the benefit and greater good of all life."

Then simply place the crystal on your own heart chakra with tip facing up and feel the full attunement for 15-20 minutes.

27   The Power Grid ~ Crystal Grid

A crystal grid, once created and charged with Reiki, will continue to send energy to heal, protect or manifest goals for up to 48 hours or longer. In addition, the Power Grid can be used as a bridge between your guides and higher self to transmit healing and help to you and your clients.

27.1 To Create a Power Grid

Carefully choose eight crystals for their intended purpose; allow your intuition to guide your selection. Clean them by placing in sea salt or sea salt water for 24 hours. Say a prayer that the crystals will be purified for the highest spiritual purpose. Create a sacred space for the grid that only you will have access to.

1. Your first step would be deciding what or whom you would like to direct this healing energy toward. After this has been decided on, you may place a picture of the person, situation, a name, or description of goal you would like to see manifested somewhere on the base of the paper for your crystal grid. The Antakarana Symbol, please see below for more information on this symbol can be drawn or represented.

2. You may also draw your Reiki symbols and their names on the underside of this paper. Be sure to say the names of the symbols 3 times and, as well, asking your Reiki guides for their support in allowing healing Reiki energy to flow through this grid for the intended purpose.

3. Choose the crystals you would like to use. Recommended is clear quartz crystal; however, follow your intuition. Attune each of the crystals to your energy and also program each one at this time toward the intended use within the grid, healing of self, healing others, manifesting goals, etc.

4. Select the crystal with the strongest yang or male energy. To be the master charging crystal suggested is a clear quartz crystal single or double pointed or one with the strongest energy as you feel guided.

5. Charge all of your crystals with Reiki. Holding each one individually at least 10 minutes empowers them with all the Reiki symbols. Invoke your spiritual guides, Reiki Masers, angels, and archangels to assist in charging and attuning your grid. You can also do a Reiki healing attunement on each crystal level III to give them an even greater charge of higher frequency energy. Once charged, place them in the grid, and don't move them. Moving weakens their energy field. Place at equal points, as shown in the diagram below. If using quartz crystals, ensure the points if any are pointing to the centre master charging crystal.

6. The remaining master crystal is to be used to keep your Power Grid charged. To do this; hold it in your dominant hand, begin drawing out the pie-shaped sections above the grid. Imagine

energy coming from the master crystal to charge the others. See diagram below to show movement between crystals.

7. As you move around the grid, repeat an affirmation/mantra or power, such as;

  •   "I charge this grid with light to heal.

  •   I charge this grid with love to heal.

  •   I call on my Reiki guides now to attune to this grid of light to heal with love."

  •   Repeat until you feel your grid is highly charged.

Feel free to use your intuitive abilities to create empowering affirmations/mantras that feel right for you.

If you have a person, project, or goal that you would like to send Reiki to, use a picture or write it on a piece of paper, and empower it will all four Reiki symbols. Hold it between your hands, empower the paper to represent your intention, and place it within your grid. Your grid will continuously send Reiki for the intended purpose.

Charge and work with your grid daily for maximum efficiency. If you can't charge the grid daily, take a picture of the grid and use your master crystal to charge the picture as a surrogate for the grid. You can place goal protection and healing work on the picture for continuous treatments.

27.2 Order of Placement of Crystals for Grid

First crystal in the red X top left.

2nd crystal on the green X top right.

3rd crystal on the blue X middle right.

4th crystal on the orange X bottom right.

Fifth crystal on the pink X bottom left.

6th crystal on the brown X middle left.

Seventh crystal on the black X in the middle with point facing the first-placed crystal in the red X.

28 Antakarana Symbol

Spelling - Antakarana or Antahkarana

In Hindu philosophy, the Antahkarana Sanskrit: "the inner cause" refers to the totality of two levels of mind, namely the Buddhi, the intellect or higher mind, and the men, the middle levels of mind, which, according to theosophy, exist as or include the mental body. Antahkarana has also been called the link between the middle and higher mind, the reincarnating part of the mind. [10]

It is a very ancient healing and meditation symbol that has been used in China and Tibet for thousands of years. The symbol is so powerful it can work independently of outside energy. The symbol interacts directly with a person's aura and chakras intuitively, as does Reiki healing energy and varies its strength according to what is required at the time and the situation.

As a healing tool, it helps to release energy in the microcosmic orbit. In the process it creates an energy flow up the main channel of the body and down the functional Channel.

The energy flow has a cleansing and grounding effect, as it activates the chakras and it heals the organs associated with each of the chakras.

_____

[10] "Antahkarana," *Wikipedia*, September 9, 2018,
https://en.wikipedia.org/w/index.php?title=Antahkarana&oldid=858731546.

29 The Healing Way

Healing is much more than overcoming illness; it is a way of life to be consciously embraced. It involves mastering oneself rather than conquering a symptom. The word healing has the same root as the words whole and holy, having to do with restoring or remembering oneness, wholeness, and holiness. Healing addresses our core, including deep psychological processes, the richness of the deep psyche and the resolution of all conflicts and relationships.

Healing is described as; the integration of body, mind, and spirit letting go of resistance; learning to love oneself fully; correcting one's relationship with God; atonement at-one-ment; remembering who one is; finding one's way home; seeking wholeness; uncovering and healing the wounds we all carry.

While there are shared stages of healing, the path is different for each person. Symbolically, we are all climbing a mountain, but there are many paths. The life that one has at this present moment is, however, one's healing path. Respecting and honouring your situation, no matter what it is, is an important aspect of healing.

Conventional thinking says that some people are well, while others need to be healed; often judging symptoms as bad, while health, wealth, and happiness are judged as well. But healing, on the other hand, is a decision or intention to become all we were created to be. The universe then conspires breathes with us to create conditions to direct one upon the path of healing. Symptoms, situations, and challenges are ways the psyche directs our actions toward healing. If we suppress a symptom or avoid a situation, often the psyche will present the lesson again in another form.

Although most healers believe that all conditions are created from within, one has the power to give away one's power and delude oneself that someone or something 'did it to them'. Taking full responsibility for whatever exists in one's life is very empowering; if you created a condition, you can uncreate it. But taking responsibility may cause extreme guilt, remorse, and self-blame, usually originating from old attitudes about a harsh, judgmental God or other harsh authority figures that have become internalized. In healing, guilt is a primary emotion to be released through forgiveness of self and others. Guilt, fears, failure, low self-worth, and so many other false beliefs are reinforced by the customs, laws, and institutions of society. The entire legal system is built upon projecting and proving blame; most of the medical system is built upon projecting blame for disease outside of ourselves.

Shifting perceptions and attitudes may be the single most important activity in which we can engage. Part of changing perspective is not to take anything too seriously; to be 'in the world but not of it.' Excessive seriousness - even about healing - slows or even stops the process. Many of us still suffer from the disease of "should-ism."

Speaking of techniques or modalities is an endless subject; the multiplicity of healing methods reflects just how complex we are. But it also reflects how exotic and remarkable is the universe of unlimited possibilities. Understanding the unlimited potential for healing facilitates healing, as it helps release the fear and despair that are often at the root of what must be overcome for healing to occur. Healing, therefore, involves an expansion of awareness. To the extent one believes in any method, it will be effective for healing. Methods are only triggering for healing and healing miracles occur quite commonly if one takes the time to look for them. i.e., raising one's awareness to what is taking place within and around them.

Healing happens! Doctors, nurses, psychologists, ministers, and others facilitate the healing process and are themselves involved in their own healing process. No one is better than another, or more 'advanced' than another; some have just developed certain gifts or are more open and able to share with others. Procedures, pills, remedies, and many other rituals are also facilitators. And who hasn't had the healing benefits of looking at a sunset, petting a favourite animal, talking to a friend, or a thousand other experiences?

We are confused today by laws that tell us that only those with licenses or that which is 'approved' can heal us. They are only silly attempts to control the healing arts. They promote false beliefs and limit healing, thus harming an unaware public. Research reports that individuals who question and even disobey their doctors, taking back control of their healing process, are far better than the 'good' cooperative patients.

Healing goes beyond the simple goal of survival of the physical body; if used as a springboard, healing teaches there may be value in suffering. Thousands of lives have been transformed by near death and out of body experiences, presenting death as a transition to another dimension, and certainly not the end of life.

For healing to truly occur, one must positively desire more energy, more enjoyment, more fulfillment or happiness in one's life. Negative desires include the avoidance of disease and death or fear of loss or of the unknown. Fear can be a stage of healing, as one realizes that one's life is not moving in the desired direction, or that something is missing. Most of the time, we are successful in ignoring it or distracting ourselves from it. A strong desire and intention for healing, no matter how it is felt, are most helpful; it is our desires that create our lives.

Healing at the deepest level is inevitable. For some, the time is now; for others, it may take many years or lifetimes. We are given the right to suffer and be miserable for as long as we wish. The process can be speeded up by asking that it proceed now, that the veils be lifted and that all the barriers to loving oneself be brought to life.

Healing can be slowed by an unwillingness to face oneself, or when one is caught in some temporary benefit of an illness or other situation. Illness or misfortune may be a way to avoid responsibility, to command attention from family or friends; to feel sorry for oneself or to avoid work.

Healing can be painful and scary. The more one is identified with the body and emotions, the worse it feels. Realizing that one is more than the physical shell is most helpful. Pain-killing drugs, although helpful under the right conditions, can block the very feelings that would lead to healing. Healing requires the willingness to feel intensely and live with passion.

Healing often involved developing discipline; as aspect of mastery of a challenge in life; from following one's own guidance, controlling the body and emotions, regiments that restrain the body and brain, following a diet, doing some exercise, or working through emotional traumas. One may indeed choose illness to learn a new discipline.

Some people understand the power of faith and prayer. True faith helps one stop worrying, fearing or being angry about one's condition; removing stress from the body and enhancing or allowing healing to proceed more rapidly. Allowing and surrender are important spiritual aspects of healing. One does not surrender to an illness, but surrenders to the higher will or God's will. One must understand that God's will is better than anything our puny egos can come up with. Often one has to exhaust one's own solutions first, and arrive at a place of utter despair. Eventually, we surrender not only our bad habits, but also our fears, despair, and feelings of smallness and insignificance. Eventually it is all placed on the altar of sacrifice and given up. Perhaps this is the ultimate goal of healing. We give up all this is not of God, and we are truly made over in his image.

Excerpted and rewritten from The Arizona Networking News, Aug/Sept 1995, vol. 14, No. 4 by Larry Wilson

30   The Dynamics of Commitment

Our desire and enthusiasm for this spiritual endeavour will stagnate is it is not focused to definite ends through a dedicated commitment. Too speedily developing in this matter would produce a confusion of efforts resulting more in chaos than character. Unless the mind is properly prepared to receive, the content - like chaff- falls upon rocky soil. Contact is not destination. It is not so much the receptor that is uppermost, as is the ability to accept, understand, and absorb that which is given. There is a deep purpose in all telepathic efforts with the etheric realms. That purpose is never one of frivolity or entertainment. Truths are needed by others to advance themselves. The equipment for advancement is truth. Truth lived and absorbed into the earth, life becomes the armour of achievement on this physical plane.

All cosmic telepathic endeavours should be entered into in the attitude of dedication to service to humanity.

In principle, the human mind is a form of energy. When in the body, each mind has a distance frequency of operation, depending on the particular characteristics of that brain which it inhabits. While we do not completely understand it, we know that it has to do with a magnetic or electrical circuit dimensions within the neurons.

Universal mind, or the mental continuum, interpenetrates all dimensions and, therefore, knows no limitations to hinder the flow of thought. The physical brain is subject to limitation of the ability of one to think, but thinking is not the act of mind; it is the activity of the cortex surrounding the outer edge of the brain.

Thought occurs within Mind, which is your higher self 0- the uniqueness that is you. It is aware of all that is happening to you and all of your thinking processes. Anything and everything in our entire universe and every dimension it encompass can be penetrated by thought, which is the Universal Life Force action within you.

It is the mind action before it is deposited into the brain thinking processes. Thought enters the tensor sector of the brain from mind. Basically, then, telepathy is communication between your Higher Self and the Higher Self of another living being. One places a thought within the other, or sends a thought to the other, where it is held in store for the thinking brain, which in turn converts the thought into something it can recognize or understand.

Keep ever before you the fact that your mind is a spiritual part of you outside your physical form, therefore outside of your brain. Brain indulges in thinking; mind brings in thought. As your ability to work with the higher mind develops, your eager mind, piercing the heights of mental awareness, will lead you into higher through emanations from great teachers in the outer universe. They anxiously await the flight of your receptive mind into their dimensions of great truth, for they are only a thought away.

Each organ of the physical body has, in turn, its own magnetic field of various frequencies, and all flows together to produce the whole in this electrical like aura, which is the soul. Each organ of the body contributes to the frequency pattern of the whole, each dependent upon the energy- the particular frequency - of the other to coordinate the uniqueness of your personal frequency. This is the principle behind the statement that illness is only a maladjustment in body frequencies, short-circuiting the whole.

All of us use a certain system is assisting the initiate on the pathway to unfolding awareness.

1. First, we lead the soul through its curiosity pursuit or the initial beginnings of telepathic exercise.

2. The we satisfy its many, many personal questions and needs.

3. Then we withdraw for a period to allow the soul to turn its attention to mental preparation; to feed the mind with knowledge and understanding books, lectures, conferences, and personal experience.

4. Then we see concentrating attention upon personal growth and development for broader use of contact.

5. Ultimately, when these preliminary stages are completed, we then approach the soul once more with the divine purpose. The purpose of all higher contact is always to call upon humans to consider the fact of spirit survival and to intelligently prepare for it with growth and understanding toward that end; and to sense the personal destiny in the incarnation, and finally to experience a deeper understanding of the greater cosmos and our relationship to all creation, in all the universal planes of existence. This is always the message, and when it is totally absorbed by the initiate, then he is ready to teach others. To help understand these approaches further, we can use certain words to further clarity:

30.1 CURIOSITY

Teachers need to hold the attention of the student at any cost - any method - contact, and not content, is the issue here. Much trivia and irrelevancy are present as the student learns to listen.

30.2 CONVICTION

Through seeking much earthly and personal information, the muddy waters of trivia begin to clear, still with a strong mixture of false and truth; until discernment takes over, while keeping pace with new revelation. Insatiable hunger for books, lectures, and like-minded people.

30.3 CONCENTRATION

Messages begin to depart the personal level and approach the character level; becoming more spiritual, more dependable, from higher sources

30.4 CONSECRATION

At this point, soul memory is triggered, fear is dispelled, and desire to truly serve is awakened, as messages enter greater depth of truth and wisdom.

30.5 COMMISSION

A certain and sure gift becomes distinctly present for the mission that soul has in service to the world

30.6 COMMITMENT

Here a sense of mission, even perhaps an awareness of its nature, flows into the soul along with the call, "Follow Me!"

Author Unknown

31 Bibliography

Bibliography:

Beacons of Change. "Reiki Attunement." (2025).